90 Days to Your Best Shape

A Science-Based Fitness Transformation

CHRIS G. WENCHELL

"You can have results or excuses, not both."

- Arnold Schwarzenegger

"Don't count the days; make the days count."

- Anderson Silva

---

90 Days to Your Best Shape: A Science-Based Fitness Transformation

I. Introduction

II. Understanding Your Body

III. Nutrition for Transformation

IV. Effective Workouts

V. Periodization and Variety

VI. Monitoring and Accountability

A. Tracking and Consistency Principles: Insights from "Bigger Leaner Stronger."
B. Tools for Tracking Progress.
C. The Importance of Accountability Partners or Communities.
D. The Role of Goal Setting in Motivation.

VII. Recovery and Rest

A. The Significance of Rest and Recovery: Insights from "Body by Science."
B. Strategies for Managing Fatigue and Injury Prevention.
C. The Role of Sleep and Stress Management.

VIII. Troubleshooting Plateaus

A. Address Common Plateaus and Obstacles.
B. Strategies to Break Through Plateaus and Stay Motivated.
C. Emotional Eating and Behavior Change.

IX. Lifestyle Considerations

A. The Role of Sleep, Stress, and Daily Habits in Fitness Success.
B. The Importance of Overall Well-Being.
C. Post-90-Day Maintenance and Long-Term Lifestyle Changes.

X. Mindset and Motivation

A. Maintaining a Positive Mindset and Staying Motivated Throughout the Journey.

XI. Injury Prevention

A. Guidance on Proper Form, Warm-Up Routines, and Injury Prevention Techniques for Workouts.

XII. Supplements

A. The Role of Supplements in Supporting Fitness Goals.

Preface

Welcome to "90 Days to Your Best Shape: A Science-Based Fitness Transformation." This book is your compass on a journey toward becoming the best version of yourself. It's a comprehensive guide to help you achieve significant results in just three months. In these pages, you'll discover the power of science-backed principles, practical strategies, and real-life inspiration to reach your peak of well-being.

The quest for better health and physical vitality is an endeavor that many of us embark upon with passion and determination. Whether you're an eager beginner or a seasoned fitness enthusiast seeking a fresh perspective, this book offers a roadmap to your destination.

The 90-day approach is not a promise of instant transformation, but a commitment to gradual and sustainable progress. It respects your individuality, acknowledges your unique starting point, and understands the challenges you face. It recognizes that success in fitness isn't determined by the finish line but by the journey you undertake—one step at a time.

This book is not a one-size-fits-all solution. Instead, it presents a blueprint for a transformation journey that is tailored to you. It combines the wisdom of some of the most influential fitness and wellness authors and thinkers, offering you a blend of science, experience, and personalization.

Within these chapters, you'll delve into the principles of nutrition, discover the secrets of effective workouts, explore the importance of mental resilience, and learn to embrace a holistic approach to well-being. You'll find practical tools, including sample meal plans, workout routines, and guidance on tracking your progress.

Moreover, you'll uncover the inspiration of real-life case studies and personal testimonials, proving that your goals are attainable.

It's worth noting that this book isn't just about the next 90 days. It's about the knowledge and habits you'll acquire to sustain your best shape for a lifetime. It's about understanding that this journey is not just about physical change, but about evolving your entire perspective on health, wellness, and self-improvement.

So, as you embark on this transformative journey, remember that each day you commit is a step closer to your best shape. You have the power within you to change, to grow, and to thrive.
Now, take a deep breath, turn the page, and let's begin the next 90 days together. Your transformation journey starts now.

Chapter I: Introduction

90 Days to Your Best Shape: A Science-Based Fitness Transformation

A. The 90-day Fitness Program Concept

Welcome to "90 Days to Your Best Shape: A Science-Based Fitness Transformation." In the next 90 days, we'll embark on a life-changing journey, one that promises to redefine your fitness, boost your confidence, and unlock the best version of yourself.

The concept is simple but powerful: within just 90 days, you can make incredible strides towards the fitness goals you've long aspired to achieve. Whether you're a fitness enthusiast or just starting your journey, this program is designed to help you maximize your potential in a focused and effective way.

B. The Target Audience for This Book

Are you passionate about fitness and relatively mindful of your dietary choices, but still find yourself battling stubborn pockets of fat that refuse to budge? If this sounds like you, you're in the right place. I've tailored this program for individuals like you, who are ready to take on the challenge of transforming their bodies and lives.

Stubborn fat can be a common nemesis for many. But you're not alone in this struggle. And with the right approach, you can overcome it. You're not just looking for minor changes; you desire significant results, and that's precisely what this program is designed to deliver.

C. The Importance of a Science-Based Approach

This program is not about fad diets, quick fixes, or unproven workout routines. It's grounded in science. I'm here to guide you through a systematic, evidence-based process that has been inspired by the insights from some of the most reputable books and experts in the field of fitness and health.

Science is our compass, helping us navigate the path to your best shape. We'll demystify the fitness journey, breaking it down into manageable steps and strategies that have been tried, tested, and proven. By understanding the science behind your transformation, you'll be better equipped to make informed decisions, and more importantly, achieve lasting results.

D. The 90-Day Challenge: An Opportunity for Transformation

Why 90 days? This timeframe is carefully chosen because it strikes the right balance between being achievable and effective. It's long enough for you to make substantial changes but short enough to maintain your focus and motivation. It's a challenge worth embracing, a commitment to yourself, and a promise of transformation.

For those of you who've already embarked on fitness journeys, you know that progress often takes time. But sometimes, we need a catalyst, a defined period where we give our absolute best to reach our goals. That's precisely what the next 90 days represent—an opportunity to give it your all, to push your limits, and to witness the remarkable changes that are within your grasp.

E. The Science-Based Approach: Your Path to Success

You might be wondering why a "science-based" approach is so crucial. Fitness and nutrition are fields with a vast amount of information and advice, not all of it reliable or effective. This program is anchored in science because it provides a structured, evidence-backed, and proven path to your goals.

We'll draw from the lessons of experts and the wisdom of scientific research to ensure every step you take is efficient and effective. No more guesswork, no more trial and error. I'll explain the "why" behind the "what" and "how," so you can approach your transformation with confidence and clarity.

With science as our guide, we'll explore the most effective ways to address common fitness challenges, including stubborn fat. We'll uncover the principles of nutrition and exercise that will unlock your potential. It's not about following a trendy diet or chasing quick fixes; it's about equipping you with knowledge and a plan that stands the test of time.

F. Your Role in This Journey

This program is a partnership, and your role is pivotal. Your commitment, dedication, and consistency are essential to your success. While I provide the roadmap and guidance, you are the driver of your journey.

Throughout the program, I'll offer you the tools, strategies, and support you need, but it's up to you to apply them. Your mindset, your determination, and your perseverance will be your greatest assets. This journey won't always be easy, but it will be worthwhile.

So, whether you're a seasoned fitness enthusiast or someone who is relatively new to the world of fitness, this program is for you. It's designed to be adaptable, catering to your unique needs, goals, and fitness level. Your transformation is personal, and this book is here to help you every step of the way.

G. What's Next

In the following chapters, we'll delve deeper into the specifics of this program. I'll help you understand your body, set personalized goals, design a nutrition plan that suits your tastes and needs, create effective workout routines, and ensure that you recover optimally. We'll also tackle the mental and emotional aspects of your transformation, offering insights into maintaining a positive mindset and staying motivated.

Your journey begins here, with your commitment and a clear understanding of the science-based principles that will propel your transformation. It won't always be easy, but it will be rewarding. By the end of this program, you'll not only see a new you in the mirror but feel a profound change in your overall well-being.

The next 90 days are yours for the taking.

Let's get started.

Chapter II: Understanding Your Body

A. The Role of Genetics and Metabolism in Stubborn Fat

Before we delve into the nitty-gritty of our 90-day fitness program, it's essential to understand the factors that contribute to stubborn fat, a common adversary for many. While genetics and metabolism play a significant role, they don't have to be insurmountable obstacles.

Genetics: The Hand You're Dealt

Genetics are like the cards you're dealt in a game of poker. They determine your baseline tendencies for body composition. Some people are naturally lean, while others may have a genetic predisposition to carry more fat in certain areas. However, your genetics do not have the final say in your fitness journey.

Understanding your genetic predispositions can help you tailor your approach and set realistic expectations. You may need to work harder in certain areas, but the right strategies can still lead to significant change.

Metabolism: The Body's Engine

Metabolism is often misunderstood. It's not just about speed; it's about how efficiently your body processes energy. Your metabolism is influenced by a variety of factors, including age, muscle mass, activity level, and more.

The key takeaway is that you can influence your metabolism through lifestyle choices. Proper nutrition and exercise play crucial roles in revving up your metabolism and burning stubborn fat.

B. The Importance of a Proper Assessment

Understanding your body and its unique characteristics is fundamental to your transformation journey. Without a clear picture of where you're starting, it's challenging to map out a path to your destination.

Assessing Your Starting Point

A proper assessment involves taking stock of various aspects of your current physical condition, such as:

1. Body Composition: Measure your body fat percentage and lean muscle mass. You can do this through tools like body composition scales, DEXA scans, or skinfold calipers.

2. Strength and Fitness Level: Evaluate your strength, flexibility, and cardiovascular fitness. Are there areas where you excel, and others where you need improvement?

3. Dietary Habits: Reflect on your current eating patterns. What are your nutritional strengths and weaknesses? Do you have any dietary restrictions or preferences?

4. Lifestyle Factors: Consider your daily routines, sleep patterns, stress levels, and time constraints. These factors significantly impact your ability to commit to a fitness program.

By assessing your starting point comprehensively, you gain insights into your unique strengths and challenges. This knowledge will guide your choices throughout the program, allowing you to set realistic goals and tailor your approach to your specific needs.

C. Genetics: A Starting Point, Not a Destination

Your genetics, like the cards dealt in a poker game, can influence your body's predisposition to fat storage and muscle development. Some individuals may seem genetically blessed with naturally lean bodies, while others may appear to struggle against stubborn fat more persistently. It's important to remember that genetics only set the stage; they don't dictate the entire story of your fitness journey.

While you may have a genetic propensity for certain body compositions, it's important to note that the environment you create through your lifestyle choices can significantly influence the outcome. Proper nutrition, targeted exercise, and lifestyle modifications can help you work with your genetic predispositions, rather than against them.

Understanding your genetic tendencies allows you to set realistic goals and focus your efforts where they'll be most effective. It can serve as a source of motivation rather than an excuse for limitations.

D. Metabolism: Your Body's Engine

Metabolism is a complex process that defines how your body utilizes the energy it receives from food. Some people have a faster metabolism, meaning their bodies efficiently burn calories, while others may have a slower metabolism that processes energy less rapidly.

Your metabolism is influenced by various factors, including age, muscle mass, activity level, and hormonal balance. The good news is that you have a degree of control over your metabolism through lifestyle choices.

Exercise, particularly strength training, can increase your muscle mass, which, in turn, can boost your metabolism. Proper nutrition also plays a significant role. Consuming the right nutrients in the right proportions can support a healthy metabolic rate.

Understanding your metabolism is crucial because it empowers you to make choices that align with your goals. By focusing on factors you can control, such as your diet and exercise routine, you can optimize your metabolism for fat loss and muscle gain.

E. The Importance of a Proper Assessment

Assessing your starting point is like establishing your coordinates on a map before embarking on a journey. It's a critical step in your transformation process.

A Holistic Approach to Assessment

A comprehensive assessment takes into account various aspects of your current condition, including your physical, nutritional, and lifestyle characteristics. Here's what you should consider:

1. Body Composition: Understanding your body's current composition, specifically the ratio of body fat to lean muscle, provides a foundation for setting fitness goals.

2. Strength and Fitness Level: Assess your current level of physical fitness, encompassing strength, flexibility, and cardiovascular endurance. Identifying your strengths and weaknesses allows you to tailor your workout routine accordingly.

3. Dietary Habits: Evaluate your dietary habits and preferences. Identify areas where your nutrition is strong and areas where you can make improvements. Are there specific dietary restrictions or preferences you need to account for?

4. Lifestyle Factors: Take stock of your daily routines, including your sleep patterns, stress levels, and time constraints. These factors can significantly influence your ability to commit to a fitness program.

By conducting a thorough assessment, you gain a 360-degree view of your current situation. This knowledge empowers you to set realistic goals, make informed choices, and design a tailored fitness program that suits your unique needs and circumstances.

Chapter III: Nutrition for Transformation

One of the cornerstones of your 90-day fitness transformation is your nutrition. It's not just about what you eat but how you eat that can significantly impact your journey. We'll start by discussing the Slow Carb Diet principles, inspired by "The 4-Hour Body" by Timothy Ferriss.

Slow Carb Diet Basics

The Slow Carb Diet is a straightforward yet powerful approach to nutrition that can help you shed fat, control your blood sugar, and maintain sustained energy levels. The key principles include:

1. Focus on Proteins: Make lean protein sources, such as poultry, lean meats, and legumes, the central component of your meals. Protein helps build and repair muscles, supports satiety, and keeps your metabolism firing.

2. Minimize Carbohydrates: Reduce your intake of processed carbs, especially sugars and refined grains. Slow carbs, like lentils, black beans, and non-starchy vegetables, are the primary sources of carbohydrates.

3. Healthy Fats: Include sources of healthy fats, such as avocados, nuts, and olive oil, in your diet. Fats are essential for overall health and can aid in nutrient absorption.

4. Avoid Dairy and Gluten: Dairy and gluten are excluded on this diet. Many people have sensitivities to these substances, and avoiding them can lead to improved digestion and reduced inflammation.

5. Regular Meals: Aim for regular meal times and eat every 3-4 hours. Consistency helps stabilize blood sugar levels and prevents overeating.

6. Cheat Day: The Slow Carb Diet includes a cheat day each week. On this day, you can enjoy foods you might have been craving. It serves both as a psychological break and can also benefit your metabolism.

B. Macronutrients and Portion Control

Beyond the Slow Carb Diet principles, it's important to understand macronutrients (carbohydrates, proteins, and fats) and the role they play in your nutrition.

1. Proteins: Proteins are the building blocks of your body. They help repair and build muscle, boost your metabolism, and keep you feeling full. Aim to include a source of protein in each meal.

2. Carbohydrates: Carbs are your body's primary energy source. Slow carbs, like whole grains and vegetables, provide sustained energy and are a better choice than fast-digesting carbs. Be mindful of portion sizes, particularly for starchy carbs.

3. Fats: Healthy fats, such as those found in avocados and nuts, support overall health and can help you feel satiated. Portion control is still important since fats are calorie-dense.

C. Sample Meal Plans and Recipes
The journey to your best shape doesn't have to be tasteless or monotonous. To help you kickstart your transformation, I've

prepared a selection of sample meal plans and delicious recipes designed to align with the Slow Carb Diet principles. These offerings serve a dual purpose: they support your nutritional needs and make your journey enjoyable.

Sample Meal Plans

When embarking on a 90-day fitness program, your nutrition plays a crucial role in achieving your desired results. To support your journey, I've put together some sample meal plans and recipes inspired by the principles of the Slow Carb Diet, as discussed in "The 4-Hour Body." These are designed to help you get started on the right track, but remember to customize them to fit your dietary preferences and requirements.

Sample Meal Plans

Day 1

Breakfast: Scrambled eggs with spinach and black beans
Lunch: Grilled chicken breast with mixed vegetables
Snack: Greek yogurt with berries
Dinner: Baked salmon with quinoa and steamed broccoli

Day 2

Breakfast: Omelette with bell peppers and avocado
Lunch: Turkey and avocado salad with vinaigrette dressing
Snack: Sliced cucumbers with hummus
Dinner: Lean ground beef stir-fry with broccoli and brown rice

Day 3

Breakfast: Greek yogurt parfait with granola and mixed berries
Lunch: Quinoa salad with chickpeas, cucumbers, and feta cheese
Snack: Sliced apples with almond butter
Dinner: Grilled shrimp with asparagus and brown rice

Day 4

Breakfast: Oatmeal with sliced bananas and a drizzle of honey
Lunch: Spinach and avocado wrap with lean turkey slices
Snack: Carrot and celery sticks with hummus
Dinner: Baked chicken breast with roasted sweet potatoes and green beans

Recipes for Success

Incorporating these principles into your meals doesn't mean sacrificing flavor. I've compiled a library of recipes that are both nutritious and delicious. From hearty breakfast options to satisfying dinners and guilt-free snacks, you'll have a variety of recipes at your disposal.

By combining these meal plans and recipes with your understanding of macronutrients and portion control, you can craft a diet that supports your goals without leaving your taste buds unsatisfied.

Recipes

Day 1

Scrambled Eggs with Spinach and Black Beans

Ingredients:

- 2 eggs
- 1/2 cup of black beans
- A handful of spinach
- Salt and pepper to taste

Instructions:

1. In a pan, lightly sauté the spinach until wilted.

2. Whisk the eggs and add them to the pan.
3. Scramble the eggs with the spinach and black beans.
4. Season with salt and pepper to taste.

Grilled Chicken Breast with Mixed Vegetables

Ingredients:

- 1 boneless, skinless chicken breast
- Assorted mixed vegetables (bell peppers, zucchini, onions)
- Olive oil, garlic, and your choice of seasonings

Instructions:

1. Marinate the chicken in olive oil, garlic, and your preferred seasonings.
2. Grill the chicken until it reaches an internal temperature of 165°F (74°C).
3. Grill the mixed vegetables until tender and lightly charred.

Day 2

Omelette with Bell Peppers and Avocado

Ingredients:

- 2 eggs
- 1/4 cup diced bell peppers (red, green, or your choice)
- 1/4 avocado, sliced
- Salt and pepper to taste

Instructions:

1. In a bowl, whisk the eggs and season with salt and pepper.
2. Heat a non-stick pan over medium heat and add a touch of oil or cooking spray.
3. Pour the whisked eggs into the pan.

4. Add diced bell peppers on one half of the omelette.
5. Once the eggs start to set, fold the other half over the peppers.
6. Cook until the omelette is firm and lightly browned.
7. Slide the omelette onto a plate and garnish with sliced avocado.

Turkey and Avocado Salad with Vinaigrette Dressing

Ingredients:

- 4 oz lean turkey slices
- 1/4 avocado, sliced
- Mixed salad greens (lettuce, spinach, arugula, etc.)
- Vinaigrette dressing (olive oil, vinegar, Dijon mustard, herbs, and spices)

Instructions:

1. Arrange the mixed salad greens on a plate.
2. Top with lean turkey slices and sliced avocado.
3. Drizzle vinaigrette dressing over the salad.

Sliced Cucumbers with Hummus

Ingredients:

- Sliced cucumbers
- Hummus (store-bought or homemade)

Instructions:

1. Wash and slice cucumbers.
2. Serve with a side of hummus for dipping.

Lean Ground Beef Stir-Fry with Broccoli and Brown Rice

Ingredients:

- 4 oz lean ground beef
- Fresh broccoli florets
- Cooked brown rice
- Stir-fry sauce (soy sauce, garlic, ginger, and optional ingredients)

Instructions:

1. In a pan, brown the lean ground beef until fully cooked.
2. Add fresh broccoli florets and stir-fry sauce.
3. Continue cooking until the broccoli is tender and the sauce is well incorporated.
4. Serve the beef and broccoli stir-fry over cooked brown rice.

Day 3

Greek Yogurt Parfait with Granola and Mixed Berries

Ingredients:

- 1 cup Greek yogurt
- 1/4 cup granola
- 1/2 cup mixed berries (strawberries, blueberries, raspberries)

Instructions:

1. In a glass or bowl, layer Greek yogurt at the bottom.
2. Add a layer of granola on top of the yogurt.
3. Add the mixed berries as the final layer.
4. Drizzle honey over the top as desired.

Quinoa Salad with Chickpeas, Cucumbers, and Feta Cheese

Ingredients:

- 1 cup cooked quinoa
- 1 can of chickpeas, drained and rinsed
- Diced cucumbers

- Cherry tomatoes, halved
- Red onions, thinly sliced
- Crumbled feta cheese
- Fresh lemon juice
- Olive oil
- Herbs and spices (e.g., parsley, oregano, salt, and pepper)

Instructions:

1. In a large bowl, combine the cooked quinoa, chickpeas, diced cucumbers, halved cherry tomatoes, and thinly sliced red onions.
2. Add crumbled feta cheese to the salad.
3. In a separate small bowl, prepare a dressing using fresh lemon juice, olive oil, herbs, and spices. Adjust the dressing to your taste.
4. Toss the salad with the dressing until all ingredients are well-coated.

Sliced Apples with Almond Butter

Ingredients:

- Sliced apples
- Almond butter

Instructions:

1. Wash and slice apples.
2. Serve with a side of almond butter for dipping.

Grilled Shrimp with Asparagus and Brown Rice

Ingredients:

- Grilled shrimp (seasoned with your choice of spices)
- Fresh asparagus spears
- Cooked brown rice

Instructions:

1. Season the shrimp with your choice of spices (e.g., lemon, garlic, and paprika).
2. Grill the shrimp until they turn pink and slightly charred.
3. Steam or grill the fresh asparagus spears until tender.
4. Serve the grilled shrimp and asparagus over cooked brown rice.

Day 4

Oatmeal with Sliced Bananas and a Drizzle of Honey

Ingredients:

- 1/2 cup of old-fashioned oats
- Sliced bananas
- Honey (for drizzling)
- Water or milk of your choice (e.g., dairy milk, almond milk)

Instructions:

1. In a saucepan, combine the oats with water or milk according to package instructions.
2. Cook the oats until they reach your preferred consistency.
3. Serve the cooked oatmeal in a bowl.
4. Top with sliced bananas and drizzle honey over the top as desired.

Spinach and Avocado Wrap with Lean Turkey Slices

Ingredients:

- Whole-grain tortilla or wrap
- Spinach leaves
- Sliced avocado
- Lean turkey slices

- Vinaigrette dressing (olive oil, vinegar, Dijon mustard, herbs, and spices)

Instructions:

1. Lay out the whole-grain tortilla.
2. Add spinach leaves, sliced avocado, and lean turkey slices.
3. Drizzle vinaigrette dressing over the ingredients.
4. Roll up the tortilla into a wrap and slice in half.

Carrot and Celery Sticks with Hummus

Ingredients:

- Carrot and celery sticks
- Hummus (store-bought or homemade)

Instructions:

1. Wash, peel, and cut carrot and celery sticks.
2. Serve with a side of hummus for dipping.

Baked Chicken Breast with Roasted Sweet Potatoes and Green Beans

Ingredients:

- Boneless, skinless chicken breast
- Sweet potatoes, peeled and cut into cubes
- Fresh green beans
- Olive oil
- Garlic, herbs, and spices of your choice

Instructions:

1. Preheat your oven to 375°F (190°C).

2. Season the chicken breast with olive oil, garlic, herbs, and spices.
3. In a baking dish, place the seasoned chicken breast along with the sweet potato cubes and fresh green beans.
4. Roast in the preheated oven until the chicken reaches an internal temperature of 165°F (74°C) and the sweet potatoes and green beans are tender.

These sample meal plans and recipes are just a starting point. Feel free to modify and create your own based on your preferences, dietary requirements, and nutritional goals. Remember, a well-balanced diet is an essential aspect of your 90-day transformation journey.

D. Meal Planning and Grocery Shopping

Meal planning and efficient grocery shopping are key to staying on track with your nutrition plan. I'll offer guidance on how to plan your meals, create a shopping list, and navigate the grocery store. This ensures that you have the right ingredients on hand, making it easier to stick to your nutrition goals.

Effective meal planning and smart grocery shopping are your allies on this transformation journey. Let's delve into the practical aspects of ensuring you have the right ingredients on hand.

Meal Planning

Meal planning allows you to structure your eating routine and ensures you have a well-balanced diet. Consider the following when planning your meals:

1. Goal Alignment: Your meals should align with your fitness goals. If your aim is fat loss, ensure a caloric deficit. If it's muscle gain, ensure you have adequate protein and overall calories.

2. Variety: Incorporate a variety of foods to ensure you receive a broad spectrum of nutrients.

3. Preparation: Plan for meals that suit your lifestyle. Quick and easy options for busy days, and more elaborate meals when you have extra time.

4. Weekly Prep: Batch cooking and prepping ingredients in advance can save you time and effort during the week.

Grocery Shopping

Efficient grocery shopping ensures you have the necessary ingredients to create your planned meals. Consider these tips for a successful grocery trip:

1. Make a List: Prepare a shopping list based on your meal plan. This prevents impulse buying and ensures you have what you need.

2. Stick to the Perimeter: The outer sections of the grocery store usually house fresh produce, lean proteins, and whole foods. These are your primary targets.

3. Read Labels: For packaged items, read labels to make informed choices. Look for low sugar, low sodium, and minimal additives.

4. Stock Up on Staples: Keep a supply of staple items like legumes, healthy fats, and whole grains so you always have a foundation for your meals.

Chapter IV: Effective Workouts

A. High-Intensity Resistance Training: Principles from "Body by Science"

As we transition into the physical aspect of your transformation, it's crucial to understand the principles of high-intensity resistance training. This method, inspired by the book "Body by Science," forms the backbone of your workout routines.

The Power of High-Intensity Training

High-Intensity Resistance Training focuses on quality over quantity. It emphasizes the following key principles:

1. Brief Workouts: The primary focus is on short, intense workouts that are time-efficient and highly effective.

2. Full-Body Workouts: High-intensity training often involves full-body exercises to maximize muscle engagement and calorie burn.

3. Progressive Overload: The workouts are designed to continually challenge your muscles, promoting growth and strength improvements.

4. Safeguarding Joint Health: By using slow and controlled movements, the risk of injury is minimized, making it accessible for all fitness levels.

B. Structured Workout Plans for All Fitness Levels

Whether you're just beginning your fitness journey or you're already well-versed in exercise, I've structured workout plans that cater to all fitness levels.

<u>Beginner</u>

- **Foundation Building:** If you're new to exercise, we'll focus on building a strong foundation. Your workouts will be shorter, less intense, and focus on perfecting your form.

<u>Intermediate</u>

- **Progressive Workouts:** As you become comfortable with the exercises, we'll gradually increase the intensity and duration of your workouts.

<u>Advanced</u>

- **Advanced Training:** For those with more experience, we'll introduce advanced techniques and exercises that challenge your strength and endurance.

C. Progressive Overload: Insights from "StrongLifts 5x5"

The concept of progressive overload is at the heart of your workout routines. It's drawn from the "StrongLifts 5x5" approach and is vital for continued muscle growth and strength development.

The Principle of Progress

Progressive overload is the practice of gradually increasing the resistance or intensity of your workouts to challenge your muscles continually. This principle is at the core of building strength and muscle, and it's vital for ongoing improvements in your fitness journey. Key elements include:

1. Strength Gains: Regularly increasing the weight you lift or the intensity of your exercises helps your body adapt, grow stronger, and build muscle over time.

2. Consistency: Consistency is the key to effective progressive overload. Regular, structured workouts and gradual increases in resistance lead to noticeable progress over time.

3. Recovery: Balancing your training with adequate rest is crucial. We'll delve into the significance of rest days, sleep, and proper nutrition for muscle recovery.

D. Detailed Sample Workout Routines

To put theory into practice, I've included a variety of detailed sample workout routines that cater to various fitness goals and levels. These routines are designed to be adaptable, whether your primary goal is fat loss, muscle gain, or overall fitness.

I've got you covered with full-body workouts, upper and lower body splits, and specialized routines that target specific areas. Each routine comes with instructions, tips on form, and recommendations for progression.

Below are sample workout routines for different fitness levels to help you get started on your 90-day transformation journey.

Sample Workout Routines

Beginner

High-Intensity Resistance Training (HIRT)

1. Leg Press: Use a leg press machine or resistance bands. Perform 1 set of 8-10 repetitions with a challenging weight.
2. Chest Press: Use a chest press machine or resistance bands. Perform 1 set of 8-10 repetitions with a challenging weight.
3. Lat Pulldown: Use a lat pulldown machine or resistance bands. Perform 1 set of 8-10 repetitions with a challenging weight.
4. Plank: Perform a plank for 30 seconds to 1 minute.

Frequency: 2-3 times per week.

Intermediate

High-Intensity Resistance Training (HIRT)

1. Leg Press: Perform 2 sets of 8-10 repetitions with a challenging weight.
2. Chest Press: Perform 2 sets of 8-10 repetitions with a challenging weight.
3. Lat Pulldown: Perform 2 sets of 8-10 repetitions with a challenging weight.
4. Overhead Press: Use a resistance band or dumbbells. Perform 2 sets of 8-10 repetitions.
5. Plank: Perform a plank for 1-2 minutes.

Frequency: 2-3 times per week.

Advanced

High-Intensity Resistance Training (HIRT)

1. Leg Press: Perform 2-3 sets of 8-10 repetitions with a challenging weight.
2. Chest Press: Perform 2-3 sets of 8-10 repetitions with a challenging weight.
3. Lat Pulldown: Perform 2-3 sets of 8-10 repetitions with a challenging weight.

4. Overhead Press: Perform 2-3 sets of 8-10 repetitions with a challenging weight.
5. Deadlift: Use a barbell. Perform 2-3 sets of 5-8 repetitions with a challenging weight.
6. Plank: Perform a plank for 2-3 minutes.

Frequency: 2-3 times per week.

Fat Loss

High-Intensity Resistance Training (HIRT) with Cardio Integration

1. Leg Press: Use a leg press machine or resistance bands. Perform 2 sets of 10-12 repetitions with a challenging weight.
2. Chest Press: Use a chest press machine or resistance bands. Perform 2 sets of 10-12 repetitions with a challenging weight.
3. Lat Pulldown: Use a lat pulldown machine or resistance bands. Perform 2 sets of 10-12 repetitions with a challenging weight.
4. High-Intensity Interval Training (HIIT): Incorporate short bursts of intense cardio exercises (e.g., sprints, jumping jacks) between resistance sets. Perform 30 seconds of high-intensity cardio followed by 30 seconds of rest.
5. Plank: Perform a plank for 1-2 minutes.

Frequency: 3-4 times per week.

Muscle Building

Progressive Overload with Compound Movements

1. Squats: Use a barbell or resistance bands. Perform 3-4 sets of 6-8 repetitions with a challenging weight.
2. Bench Press: Use a barbell or dumbbells. Perform 3-4 sets of 6-8 repetitions with a challenging weight.
3. Bent-Over Rows: Use a barbell or dumbbells. Perform 3-4 sets of 6-8 repetitions with a challenging weight.

4. Deadlift: Use a barbell. Perform 3-4 sets of 5-6 repetitions with a challenging weight.

5. Pull-Ups: Perform 3-4 sets of 6-8 repetitions (use assistance or resistance bands if needed).

6. Rest: Allow adequate rest between sets to maximize strength and muscle gains.

Frequency: 3-4 times per week.

Endurance and Cardiovascular

Cardiovascular Training with Varied Intensity

1. Running: Go for a 30-45 minute run at a moderate pace on one day.

2. Cycling: Cycle for 45-60 minutes at a steady pace on another day.

3. Interval Training: Perform interval training with bursts of high-intensity exercise (e.g., sprinting, jump rope) for 20-30 seconds followed by 30 seconds of rest, repeating 5-8 times on a different day.

4. Swimming: Swim for 30-45 minutes at a steady pace on another day.

5. Hiking: Plan a 2-3 hour hike in a natural setting to improve endurance and enjoy the outdoors.

Frequency: 4-5 times per week.

These sample workout routines are designed to provide structure and guidance based on your fitness level. However, it's essential to tailor your workouts to your individual goals, preferences, and any specific needs or restrictions you may have. Remember that progressive overload, challenging yourself with each workout, is a key principle for achieving significant results in your 90-day fitness program.

Chapter V: Periodization and Variety

Your fitness journey is an ongoing process, and variety in your workouts is a vital component for continued progress. We draw inspiration from programs like P90X to emphasize the significance of workout variety.

The Benefits of Variety

1. Muscle Confusion: Constantly changing your workouts keeps your muscles guessing and prevents adaptation. This muscle confusion leads to better results and minimizes plateaus.

2. Mental Engagement: Variety keeps your workouts exciting and mentally engaging, reducing the risk of boredom and maintaining motivation.

3. Balanced Development: Different workouts target various muscle groups and energy systems, ensuring balanced development and overall fitness.

4. Injury Prevention: Changing your routine can help prevent overuse injuries and reduce the risk of chronic strain.

B. The Role of Periodization in Preventing Plateaus

As your fitness level improves, you may encounter plateaus where progress seems to stall. This is where the concept of periodization comes into play.

What Is Periodization?

Periodization is the structured variation of intensity, volume, and exercise selection in your training program. It involves dividing your workouts into cycles, with each cycle having specific goals and intensity levels.

The primary components of periodization include:

1. Microcycles: Short-term periods (typically one to four weeks) that focus on specific training goals and variations.

2. Mesocycles: Medium-term periods (usually several months) that encompass a series of microcycles and work towards a broader training objective, such as strength or endurance.

3. Macrocycles: Long-term plans (usually a year or more) that consist of multiple mesocycles and facilitate the achievement of your ultimate fitness goals.

Preventing Plateaus

By incorporating periodization into your training plan, you can effectively prevent plateaus and experience continuous improvement. The variations in intensity, volume, and exercises challenge your body in different ways, ensuring that it never fully adapts to a routine. This helps you break through stagnant phases and keeps your progress on track.

Chapter VI: Monitoring and Accountability

In the pursuit of your best shape, tracking your progress and maintaining consistency are paramount. We draw inspiration from principles found in "Bigger Leaner Stronger" to explore these vital aspects of your fitness journey.

The Power of Tracking

1. Measurement Motivates: Regularly measuring and tracking your progress, whether it's weight, body measurements, or workout performance, provides motivation by showcasing your improvements.

2. Identifying Plateaus: Tracking helps you spot plateaus early. When you notice a stagnation in your progress, it's a signal to reassess your approach and make necessary adjustments.

3. Setting Realistic Goals: It's easier to set and achieve realistic goals when you have accurate data. Tracking helps you create milestones that are both challenging and attainable.

B. Tools for Tracking Progress

In the digital age, various tools and technologies can aid in tracking your fitness progress. From workout logs to dedicated apps, you have an array of options at your disposal.

1. Workout Logs: Traditional workout logs allow you to document your exercises, weights, reps, and sets. They provide a tangible record of your workouts and can be valuable for identifying trends.

2. Fitness Apps: Many mobile apps are designed to help you track workouts, nutrition, and progress. These apps often include features like workout plans, calorie counting, and social support.

3. Wearable Devices: Wearable fitness trackers and smartwatches can monitor your activity, heart rate, and even sleep patterns. These devices provide real-time data and insights into your daily habits.

C. The Importance of Accountability Partners or Communities

Accountability is a powerful force in maintaining consistency and motivation throughout your fitness journey.

1. Accountability Partners: A workout buddy or an accountability partner can be a valuable source of motivation. Sharing your goals and progress with someone else creates a sense of responsibility, encouraging you to stay on track. You can schedule workouts together, discuss challenges, and celebrate victories, creating a supportive environment that bolsters your commitment.

2. Online Communities: Joining online fitness communities, social media groups, or forums allows you to connect with like-minded individuals. Sharing your journey and hearing about the experiences of others can inspire and encourage you. It provides a sense of belonging, and the exchange of advice and support can be invaluable. Whether you're seeking advice on nutrition, discussing workout routines, or sharing your accomplishments, the sense of community fosters a powerful sense of accountability.

D. The Role of Goal Setting in Motivation

Setting clear and meaningful goals is a crucial aspect of your fitness journey, providing direction and motivation.

1. Short-Term vs. Long-Term Goals: Establish both short-term and long-term goals. Short-term goals provide regular checkpoints for progress, while long-term goals help maintain your overall vision. Short-term goals might include reaching a certain weight or running a specific distance within a month, while long-term goals could encompass achieving your ideal body composition over a year.

2. SMART Goals: Use the SMART criteria (Specific, Measurable, Achievable, Relevant, Time-bound) when setting goals. This framework ensures your goals are well-defined and attainable. For example, a SMART goal might be "Lose 10 pounds in 3 months by following a specific diet and exercise plan."

3. Visualizing Success: Regularly visualize your success. Create a mental image of what achieving your goals will look and feel like. Visualizing your ideal self, the activities you'll be able to enjoy, and the confidence you'll exude can be a powerful motivational tool. This mental picture serves as a reminder of what you're working toward.

4. Rewarding Achievements: Celebrate your accomplishments. Recognize and reward your efforts to maintain a positive outlook and stay motivated. These rewards can be non-food related, such as buying new workout gear, treating yourself to a spa day, or taking a weekend trip.

Chapter VII: Recovery and Rest

A. The Significance of Rest and Recovery: Insights from "Body by Science"

In your journey toward your best shape, rest and recovery are not mere luxuries; they are critical components. We draw inspiration from principles found in "Body by Science" to emphasize the importance of recovery.

The Restorative Power of Rest

1. Muscle Repair and Growth: During rest, your body repairs and rebuilds muscles damaged during exercise. This process is essential for muscle growth and strength development.

2. Injury Prevention: Adequate rest reduces the risk of overuse injuries and chronic strain. It allows your joints and muscles to recover and prepares them for future challenges.

3. Energy Restoration: Rest replenishes your energy stores, including glycogen levels, which are crucial for fueling your workouts and daily activities.

4. Mental Rejuvenation: Rest is equally important for your mental health. It helps reduce stress, improve focus, and maintain motivation.

B. Strategies for Managing Fatigue and Injury Prevention

Fatigue and injuries can be significant roadblocks in your fitness journey. Employing effective strategies can help you manage these challenges.

1. Listen to Your Body: Pay attention to your body's signals. If you experience persistent fatigue, soreness, or discomfort, it's a sign that you might need more rest or a change in your workout routine.

2. Periodization: Periodize your training plan to include lighter phases. These recovery periods allow your body to recuperate, reducing the risk of overtraining and injuries.

3. Active Recovery: Engage in active recovery, which involves low-intensity activities like walking, swimming, or yoga. Active recovery promotes blood flow, aiding in the repair of muscles and the removal of waste products.

C. The Role of Sleep and Stress Management

Sleep and stress are often underestimated factors in fitness, yet they play a vital role in your progress.

1. Sleep: Quality sleep is essential for recovery. During deep sleep, your body releases growth hormone, critical for muscle repair and growth. Aim for 7-9 hours of uninterrupted sleep per night.

2. Stress Management: High stress levels can hinder your progress by elevating cortisol, a hormone that promotes fat storage and muscle breakdown. Employ stress management techniques such as meditation, deep breathing, or engaging in hobbies to relax and reduce stress. These practices help you maintain a positive mindset and overall well-being, which are crucial for your fitness journey.

Chapter VIII: Troubleshooting Plateaus

In any fitness journey, plateaus and obstacles are bound to arise. Identifying and understanding these common challenges is the first step in overcoming them.

Common Plateaus

1. Weight Plateaus: After initial weight loss, you might find your progress stagnating. This is a common plateau caused by your body adapting to a new caloric intake.

2. Strength Plateaus: As you become stronger, there may come a point where you struggle to increase the weight you lift or the number of repetitions you perform.

3. Motivational Plateaus: At times, you may lose motivation, and your enthusiasm wanes. Plateaus can be as much about psychological hurdles as they are about physical ones.

B. Strategies to Break Through Plateaus and Stay Motivated

Overcoming plateaus and staying motivated are essential to reaching your best shape. Employing effective strategies can help you navigate these challenges.

1. Periodization and Variation: Continue to employ periodization techniques to change your workout routine. Variation in exercises, intensity, and rep schemes can stimulate progress.

2. Nutritional Adjustments: If you've hit a weight plateau, reevaluate your nutritional plan. Adjust your caloric intake and macronutrient ratios to break through.

3. Rest and Recovery: Ensure you're getting sufficient rest to avoid burnout. Sometimes, a period of active recovery or a week off can rejuvenate your motivation and physical performance.

4. Goal Revision: Revisit and possibly revise your goals. Sometimes your initial goals may no longer align with your current motivations or circumstances. Set new objectives that inspire you.

C. Addressing Emotional Eating and Behavior Change

Emotional eating and behavioral patterns can hinder your fitness journey. Understanding and addressing these aspects is crucial for long-term success.

Emotional Eating

Recognizing and addressing emotional eating is essential for your overall well-being and fitness progress. Here are strategies to help:

- **Mindful Eating:** Practice mindful eating, which involves paying full attention to the sensory experience of eating. It can help you become more aware of emotional triggers for overeating.

- **Emotion Management:** Develop alternative strategies for coping with emotions other than eating. This might involve engaging in physical activity, meditation, journaling, or seeking emotional support from friends, family, or a therapist.

- **Food Journaling:** Keeping a food journal can help you identify patterns of emotional eating. By recording what you eat and how you feel when you eat, you can gain insights into your behaviors.

Behavior Change

Changing habits and behaviors is often challenging but necessary for lasting transformation. Here are steps to guide you through the process:

- **Gradual Changes:** Implement gradual changes in your daily routines and habits. Trying to change too much at once can be overwhelming and lead to relapse. Small, consistent adjustments are more sustainable.

- **Consistency:** Make choices that consistently align with your fitness goals. It's the cumulative effect of these choices that leads to significant change.

- **Support and Counseling:** Seeking support from friends, family, or a therapist can be invaluable. A supportive network can provide encouragement and accountability, and professional counseling can help address underlying emotional issues that drive certain behaviors.

Chapter IX: Lifestyle Considerations

A. The Role of Sleep, Stress, and Daily Habits in Fitness Success

To achieve and maintain your best shape, it's essential to consider various lifestyle factors that impact your success, beyond diet and exercise.

Sleep

Quality sleep is the foundation of physical and mental well-being. Adequate sleep:

- **Promotes Recovery:** During deep sleep, your body undergoes essential repair and growth processes.

- **Regulates Hormones:** Sleep helps balance hormones responsible for hunger, appetite, and stress.

- **Enhances Cognitive Function:** A well-rested mind is more focused, motivated, and capable of making healthy choices.

Stress

Stress management is crucial for maintaining your fitness journey. Chronic stress can lead to:

- **Increased Fat Storage:** High stress levels can elevate cortisol, promoting fat storage and muscle breakdown.

- **Reduced Motivation:** Stress can hinder your ability to stay motivated and adhere to your fitness plan.

- **Negative Eating Habits:** Stress often leads to emotional eating, making it harder to maintain a balanced diet.

Daily Habits

Your daily habits play a significant role in your fitness success. Consider:

- **Physical Activity:** Consistent physical activity beyond structured workouts, such as walking, taking the stairs, or engaging in active hobbies.

- **Nutrition Habits:** The choices you make daily regarding food and portion control.

- **Hydration:** Staying well-hydrated supports overall health and aids in digestion and energy levels.

B. The Importance of Overall Well-Being

Your fitness journey is not just about appearance or performance; it's about overall well-being.

Mental Health

Your mental health is intrinsically linked to your physical health. Engage in practices like mindfulness, meditation, and relaxation techniques to manage stress and improve mental well-being.

Emotional Well-Being

Embrace self-compassion and self-acceptance. A positive relationship with yourself is as vital as achieving external fitness goals.

Social Connections

Maintain a supportive network of friends and family. Social connections can provide emotional support and motivation.

C. Post-90-Day Maintenance and Long-Term Lifestyle Changes

As you approach the end of your 90-day fitness journey, it's crucial to consider the long-term perspective. Maintenance and sustainable lifestyle changes are key to ensuring your hard work pays off over time.

Periodic Assessments

Regularly assess your progress to ensure you're on the right track. These assessments can help you fine-tune your approach, make necessary adjustments, and set new goals based on your evolving needs and aspirations.

Adaptation

Understand that your fitness journey is a dynamic process. There will be changes, setbacks, and fluctuations in your motivation and progress. Embrace these shifts as part of the journey, and don't be discouraged by temporary plateaus or challenges.

Integration

The principles and habits you've learned during your 90-day program should become integrated into your daily life. This encompasses not just exercise and nutrition but also factors like sleep, stress management, and mental well-being. These should be woven into your lifestyle to ensure your long-term health and fitness.

Setting New Goals

Continue to set new fitness goals. Having something to strive for keeps you motivated and engaged in your fitness journey. These goals can be related to strength, endurance, flexibility, or any aspect of fitness that resonates with you.

Chapter X: Mindset and Motivation

A. Maintaining a Positive Mindset and Staying Motivated

As you approach the conclusion of your 90-day fitness journey, it's crucial to nurture a positive mindset and maintain motivation for the long haul. Your mental outlook and motivation are powerful determinants of your fitness success.

Self-Reflection

Take a moment to reflect on how far you've come during your 90-day fitness program. Celebrate your achievements, whether they are in the form of weight loss, increased strength, improved endurance, or simply adopting healthier habits.

Gratitude

Practicing gratitude can foster a positive mindset. Focus on the positive aspects of your fitness journey and life in general. Acknowledge the support you've received and the progress you've made.

Revisiting Your "Why"

Remind yourself of the reasons you embarked on this journey. Whether it was to improve your health, gain confidence, or enhance your quality of life, reconnect with your initial motivations. Knowing your "why" can reignite your motivation.

Goal Setting

Set new goals that continue to inspire you. Having clear, achievable objectives keeps your motivation high. Consider both short-term and long-term goals to provide ongoing purpose.

Positive Self-Talk

Challenge negative self-talk and self-doubt. Replace self-criticism with positive affirmations and self-encouragement. Believing in your ability to succeed is a powerful motivator.

Visualization

Visualize your future self, living your best shape. This mental picture can motivate and inspire you to stay on track.

Surround Yourself with Positivity

Engage with a supportive community or network of friends who share your fitness aspirations. Positive, like-minded individuals can provide invaluable encouragement and motivation.

Track Your Progress

Continue to track your progress, acknowledging your achievements. This tangible evidence of your success reinforces your motivation.

Adapt to Change

Your fitness journey is a dynamic process with ups and downs. Embrace change, adapt to setbacks, and use them as opportunities to grow and learn.

Accountability and Support

Continue to lean on your accountability partners and support network. These connections provide encouragement and help keep you motivated.

Celebrate Small Wins

Don't wait for major milestones to celebrate. Recognize and celebrate small victories along the way. These achievements provide a continuous sense of accomplishment.

Stay Informed

Stay curious and engaged in your fitness journey. Keep learning about new workout techniques, nutrition, and health-related topics. Staying informed and updated keeps your journey exciting and fresh.

Recognize Plateaus as Opportunities

When you encounter plateaus, view them as opportunities for growth. These moments are when you can refine your approach, learn more about your body, and discover new strategies for success.

Be Kind to Yourself

Understand that you are human, and setbacks or moments of low motivation are normal. Be kind to yourself and avoid self-criticism. Instead, focus on self-compassion and resilience.

Embrace Enjoyable Activities

Engage in physical activities you enjoy. Whether it's dancing, hiking, or playing a sport, having fun while being active can boost your motivation and make fitness a joyful part of your life.

Conclusion

Your 90-day fitness journey is an impressive achievement, but it's not the end of the road. It's a milestone in a lifelong quest for better health and well-being. A positive mindset, unwavering motivation, and a commitment to self-improvement are your constant companions on this journey.

Chapter XI: Injury Prevention

In your ongoing fitness journey, preventing injuries is paramount. Understanding and implementing proper form, effective warm-up routines, and injury prevention techniques are key components of a safe and successful fitness regimen.

Proper Form

Maintaining proper form during exercises is essential for preventing injuries. Here are guidelines to ensure you're using correct form:

- **Education:** Learn the correct form for each exercise. This may involve watching tutorials, consulting a personal trainer, or using mirrors to monitor your form.

- **Start Light:** When introducing a new exercise, start with a lighter weight to focus on form before increasing intensity.

- **Mind-Muscle Connection:** Pay attention to the muscles being engaged during each exercise. Mindful awareness helps maintain proper form.

- **Listen to Your Body:** If you experience pain or discomfort while exercising, stop immediately and reassess your form. Ignoring discomfort can lead to injury.

Warm-Up Routines

Warming up is a crucial component of injury prevention. A proper warm-up:

- **Increases Blood Flow:** Warming up gradually increases blood flow to your muscles, preparing them for more intense activity.

- **Boosts Joint Lubrication:** It enhances joint lubrication, making movements smoother and reducing the risk of joint-related injuries.

- **Primes Your Nervous System:** A warm-up helps "wake up" your nervous system, improving the coordination of muscle contractions.

Effective warm-up routines might include light cardiovascular exercises like jogging or jumping jacks, dynamic stretching, and mobility exercises. Spend 5-10 minutes warming up before your workouts.

Injury Prevention Techniques

Incorporate injury prevention techniques into your fitness routine to minimize the risk of common workout-related injuries:

- **Strength and Flexibility Training:** Develop both strength and flexibility, as imbalances can lead to injuries. Yoga and stretching exercises are excellent complements to resistance training.

- **Rest and Recovery:** Give your muscles time to recover between intense workouts. Overtraining increases the risk of injuries.

- **Proper Footwear and Equipment:** Wear appropriate footwear and use the right equipment for your workouts. Ill-fitting shoes or equipment can contribute to injuries.

- **Listen to Your Body:** Pay attention to your body's signals. If you experience persistent discomfort or pain, don't push through it. Rest and seek professional guidance if necessary.

Gradual Progression

Gradually increase the intensity and volume of your workouts. Sudden jumps in weight or training volume can stress your muscles and joints, increasing the risk of injury.

Cross-Training

Engage in cross-training by incorporating a variety of exercises and activities. This approach prevents overuse injuries and imbalances by working different muscle groups.

Professional Guidance

If you're new to exercise or have specific health concerns, consider seeking guidance from a fitness professional, such as a personal trainer or physical therapist. They can help you develop safe and effective workout routines.

Cool-Down

After your workout, include a cool-down period. This typically involves light cardio or static stretching. Cooling down helps lower your heart rate and reduce muscle tension.

Stay Hydrated

Dehydration can contribute to muscle cramps and fatigue, increasing the risk of injury. Ensure you're adequately hydrated before, during, and after your workouts.

Nutrient Support

Maintain a balanced diet to support muscle recovery and injury prevention. Proper nutrition ensures your body has the nutrients it needs to repair and strengthen tissues.

Professional Evaluation

If you've had a previous injury or are concerned about a specific aspect of your fitness routine, consider a professional evaluation. A physical therapist or sports medicine specialist can assess your condition and provide tailored advice.

Conclusion

Injury prevention is a fundamental aspect of your fitness journey. By mastering proper form, incorporating effective warm-up routines, and embracing injury prevention techniques, you are taking proactive steps to safeguard your well-being. Remember that a consistent and safe approach to fitness is the key to a lifetime of health and vitality.

Chapter XII: Supplements

A. The Role of Supplements in Supporting Fitness Goals

Supplements can play a supplementary role in your fitness journey, but it's essential to understand their place and purpose within the broader context of a balanced diet and fitness program.

Supplementary Nature

Supplements are meant to complement, not replace, a well-balanced diet. They are designed to fill specific nutritional gaps and address individual needs.

Nutritional Gaps

Supplements can be beneficial when you have difficulty obtaining essential nutrients from food alone. For instance, individuals with specific dietary restrictions or nutrient deficiencies may benefit from supplementation.

Supporting Fitness Goals

Certain supplements can support specific fitness goals, such as muscle recovery, energy levels, or overall health. For example:

- **Protein Supplements:** Can help meet protein needs, particularly for those with high protein requirements, like athletes or bodybuilders.

- **Creatine:** May enhance strength and performance during high-intensity workouts.

- **Multivitamins:** Can fill micronutrient gaps and support overall health.

- **Omega-3 Fatty Acids:** Can reduce inflammation and support joint health, important for physically active individuals.

Consultation

Before incorporating supplements, consider consulting with a healthcare professional or registered dietitian. They can assess your specific needs and help you choose supplements that align with your fitness goals and overall health.

Safety and Quality

Choose reputable brands and products with third-party testing for quality and purity. Ensuring the safety and effectiveness of supplements is crucial.

Whole Foods

Remember that whole, natural foods should be your primary source of nutrients. Supplements should only be used when there's a specific need or deficiency that cannot be adequately addressed through dietary choices.

Targeted Supplementation

Consider supplements that specifically address your individual fitness goals. For example, if your focus is on endurance, you might explore supplements like branched-chain amino acids (BCAAs) or nitric oxide boosters. Tailoring supplementation to your goals can enhance their effectiveness.

Timing and Dosage

Pay attention to the timing and dosage of supplements. Some, like protein, are best consumed before or after workouts for optimal results. Dosage recommendations can vary, so follow guidelines provided on the supplement label or as advised by a healthcare professional.

Potential Side Effects

Be aware of potential side effects. Some supplements may have adverse effects or interact with medications you're taking. It's essential to discuss potential interactions with a healthcare provider, particularly if you have underlying health conditions.

Transparency and Labeling

Look for transparent labeling on supplements, including a list of ingredients and their amounts. Avoid supplements with proprietary blends or vague ingredient descriptions.

Personalized Approach

Your supplementation needs are highly individualized. What works for one person may not work for another. Experimentation and monitoring your body's response to supplements can help you determine what best supports your fitness goals.

Conclusion

Supplements can indeed play a supportive role in your fitness journey, but it's crucial to approach them with knowledge, caution, and a focus on their supplementary nature. By making informed choices and consulting professionals when necessary, you can harness the benefits of supplements while maintaining a balanced and nutritious diet.

Chapter XIII: Customization

A. The Importance of Personalizing the Fitness Program

In your quest for your best shape, one size does not fit all. Personalizing your fitness program is a fundamental principle that ensures your journey is tailored to your unique needs and preferences.

Individual Needs

Recognize that each individual has distinct needs, capabilities, and limitations. What works for one person may not be suitable for another. This highlights the importance of customizing your fitness approach.

Goals and Priorities

Your fitness goals and priorities are unique to you. Whether it's weight loss, muscle gain, improved endurance, or enhanced flexibility, your program should align with your aspirations.

Adaptability

A customized program is adaptable to your changing circumstances. Life can be unpredictable, and your fitness routine should be flexible enough to accommodate variations in your schedule and energy levels.

Personal Preferences

Your fitness program should reflect activities and exercises you enjoy. Incorporating exercises and routines that you find pleasurable increases the likelihood that you'll remain committed to your fitness journey.

Health Considerations

Individual health considerations are a critical aspect of customization. If you have preexisting medical conditions or specific dietary needs, these should be factored into your fitness plan.

Progress Tracking

Customization also involves tracking your progress. Monitoring your achievements, challenges, and adjustments is integral to refining and optimizing your fitness program.

Seek Professional Guidance

When creating a personalized fitness program, don't hesitate to seek professional guidance. Fitness trainers, dietitians, and healthcare providers can offer expert insights to ensure your program aligns with your unique needs and goals.

Continuous Assessment

Recognize that personalization is an ongoing process. Regularly assess and reevaluate your fitness program to ensure it remains aligned with your changing needs and aspirations.

Feedback and Self-Reflection

Actively seek feedback from yourself and others involved in your fitness journey. Self-reflection and feedback from trainers, friends, or workout partners can offer valuable insights for program customization.

Consistency

While customization allows for variety and adaptability, it's essential to maintain consistency in your fitness program. Consistency fosters progress and helps you achieve your long-term goals.

Lifestyle Integration

Customization extends beyond exercise and nutrition. It should integrate with your lifestyle, accommodating your work, family, and social commitments. This ensures that your fitness program is sustainable.

Long-Term Vision

Keep your long-term vision in mind. Your personalized fitness program should not be geared solely toward short-term results but should promote lasting health and well-being.

Celebrate Individuality

Embrace the diversity of fitness journeys and celebrate your individuality. What works for you may not work for someone else, and that's perfectly fine. Recognize and appreciate your unique path.

Conclusion

Personalization is the cornerstone of a successful and sustainable fitness journey. By recognizing and celebrating your individuality, continuously assessing and adapting your program, and integrating it into your lifestyle, you're taking steps toward achieving your best shape while enjoying the process.

Chapter XIV: Case Studies and Personal Testimonials

A. Real-Life Examples and Case Studies

The stories of real individuals and their transformative journeys can inspire and provide valuable insights for your own pursuit of your best shape. Here, we present diverse case studies and personal testimonials that highlight the power of dedication, customization, and personalization in the realm of fitness.

The Weight Loss Success Story

- Meet Sarah, a working mother who decided to take charge of her health. Through a personalized fitness program that accommodated her busy schedule, Sarah not only shed excess weight but also gained newfound confidence. Her story underscores the importance of setting realistic goals and designing a fitness program tailored to individual lifestyles.

The Strength and Endurance Breakthrough

- David, a 40-year-old professional, shares his journey of going from a sedentary lifestyle to conquering marathons. His case study emphasizes the transformative power of consistency, gradual progression, and adapting to the changing needs of your body as you age.

The Holistic Health Transformation

- Meet Lily, a young student who struggled with stress and irregular eating habits. Her journey toward her best shape focused not only on physical fitness but also mental and emotional well-being. Lily's story reminds us that holistic health is an essential component of a successful fitness program.

The Post-Injury Comeback

- John's case study is a testament to resilience. After a serious injury, he embarked on a rehabilitation journey, demonstrating that customization isn't just for beginners but can also be a lifeline for those recovering from injuries. His story highlights the significance of seeking professional guidance and tailoring workouts to address specific health considerations.

The Senior Fitness Inspiration

- Helen, at the age of 70, proves that it's never too late to embark on a fitness journey. Her case study showcases the importance of adapting workouts to accommodate age-related changes and maintaining a positive mindset to overcome challenges.

The Diverse Pathways to Success

These case studies and personal testimonials underscore that there's no one-size-fits-all approach to fitness. Each journey is unique and can be adapted to individual needs, preferences, and circumstances. The common thread among these stories is the unwavering commitment to personalization and customization.

The Postpartum Triumph

- Lisa's journey through postpartum fitness highlights the unique challenges women face after childbirth. Her case study reveals the importance of postpartum care and a customized fitness program that addresses the specific needs of new mothers.

The Weightlifting Champion

- Mark's story takes us through his journey from an average fitness enthusiast to a competitive weightlifter. His case study emphasizes how focused training and personalization can help individuals excel in their chosen fitness discipline.

The Transformation After Illness

- Sarah's case study narrates her remarkable transformation after battling a severe illness. Her journey highlights the role of fitness and nutrition in recovery and regaining overall health.

The Mental Health Reclamation

- Jake's experience focuses on the intersection of fitness and mental health. He shares how a customized fitness routine and mindfulness practices became essential tools in managing stress, anxiety, and depression.

The Lifelong Learner

- Veronica's journey reflects her commitment to continuous learning in fitness. Her case study underscores that curiosity and adaptability are key in maintaining lifelong well-being.

The Family's Fitness Odyssey

- The Smith family's collective fitness journey demonstrates how customization can be applied to accommodate various age groups and fitness levels within a family, fostering a culture of health and togetherness.

Conclusion

These diverse case studies and personal testimonials serve as a testament to the transformative power of personalization and customization in fitness journeys. The stories of these individuals from various walks of life reveal that there is no single path to your best shape.

Chapter XV: Safety Considerations

A. The Importance of Consulting with Healthcare Professionals

Before embarking on any fitness program, it's essential to prioritize your health and safety. This chapter emphasizes the critical role of consulting with healthcare professionals, particularly for individuals with underlying health conditions.

The First Step

Your journey to your best shape begins with a crucial step: consulting with a healthcare professional. Whether you're a fitness novice or an experienced enthusiast, seeking professional guidance ensures that your fitness program aligns with your unique health requirements.

Underlying Health Conditions

If you have underlying health conditions, such as heart disease, diabetes, high blood pressure, or orthopedic issues, consulting with a healthcare provider is even more paramount. They can evaluate your specific health concerns and help tailor your fitness program to accommodate these conditions.

Medications and Supplements

Healthcare professionals can assess how any medications you are taking might interact with exercise, and they can offer guidance on
the use of supplements if necessary. Understanding these interactions is crucial to your safety and well-being.

Stress Testing

In some cases, healthcare providers may recommend stress testing or other evaluations to gauge your cardiovascular health before you begin an exercise program. These assessments provide insights into your body's readiness for physical activity.

Customization for Health

Healthcare professionals can provide recommendations for exercises and routines that accommodate your health conditions while still working toward your fitness goals. This level of customization helps ensure your safety throughout your fitness journey.

Monitoring and Reporting

Your healthcare provider can also help establish a plan for monitoring your progress and addressing any issues that arise during your fitness program. Open communication with your healthcare team is vital to your safety.

Health and Fitness Assessment

A comprehensive health and fitness assessment by a healthcare provider can establish a baseline for your fitness journey. This assessment can include blood pressure checks, cholesterol evaluations, glucose monitoring, and musculoskeletal examinations, among other things.

Lifestyle and Behavior Counseling

Healthcare professionals can offer lifestyle and behavior counseling that goes beyond exercise and nutrition. They can guide you on stress management, sleep improvement, and other factors that contribute to your overall well-being.

Progress Evaluation

Throughout your fitness journey, healthcare providers can conduct periodic evaluations to track your progress and make necessary adjustments to your program. This proactive approach safeguards your health and ensures that your program remains effective.

Injury and Symptom Management

In the event of injuries, discomfort, or concerning symptoms, healthcare professionals can provide guidance on management and rehabilitation. Their expertise ensures that you address health issues promptly and safely.

Long-Term Health Goals

Consult with your healthcare provider to establish long-term health goals that align with your fitness journey. This ensures that your program supports not only short-term fitness outcomes but also sustained well-being.

Conclusion

Your health and safety are non-negotiable aspects of your fitness journey. By consulting with healthcare professionals, you're taking a proactive step to ensure that your program is tailored to your individual health needs and circumstances.

Chapter XVI: Conclusion

A. Summarizing Key Lessons

As we wrap up this comprehensive guide, it's crucial to revisit the key lessons and insights derived from both the recommended books and the 90-day fitness program. These core takeaways form the foundation for your journey to your best shape:

- **Customization and Personalization:** Your fitness journey is uniquely yours. Tailoring your program to your individual needs, preferences, and health considerations is fundamental.

- **Consultation with Healthcare Professionals:** Safety should be a priority. Consulting with healthcare professionals, especially if you have underlying health conditions, is essential to ensure a safe and effective fitness program.

- **Diverse Case Studies:** Real-life case studies and personal testimonials illustrate the transformative power of dedication, customization, and personalization in fitness journeys. There is no one-size-fits-all path to success.

- **Long-Term Vision:** Your fitness journey is not a sprint but a lifelong commitment to well-being. Maintaining a long-term vision and consistently adjusting your program is key to lasting success.

- **Nutrition and Exercise Synergy:** Both nutrition and exercise play vital roles in achieving your best shape. A balanced diet and tailored workout routines work together to enhance your fitness journey.

- **Customized Workout Plans:** Create workout plans that accommodate your fitness level, preferences, and goals. Whether it's strength training, cardiovascular workouts, flexibility exercises, or a combination, your program should reflect your unique needs.

- **Mental Resilience:** Building mental resilience is just as important as physical strength. Stay motivated, persevere through challenges, and maintain a positive mindset. The mental aspect of your fitness journey is a powerful driver of success.

- **Holistic Well-Being:** Remember that your health extends beyond physical fitness. Prioritize sleep, stress management, and overall well-being. A holistic approach ensures that you're not only in great physical shape but also leading a fulfilling and balanced life.

B. Encouragement to Begin Your Journey

With the knowledge and insights gained from this guide, it's time to embark on your own 90-day transformation journey. Remember that your path will be unique, just like the individuals in the case studies. Whether your goal is weight loss, strength gain, improved endurance, or holistic well-being, your dedication and customization are your greatest allies.

Now that you have the tools, knowledge, and inspiration, it's time to take action. Your 90-day transformation journey is a chance to redefine your well-being and achieve your best shape. Don't wait for the "perfect" moment; start today. Every small step you take is a move in the right direction.

Remember, progress is not always linear. You may face setbacks and challenges, but each one is an opportunity for growth. Stay committed to your vision and trust in the customization and personalization principles that guide your path.

C. Resources and Tools for Ongoing Support

To support your journey, consider the following resources and tools:

- **Professional Guidance:** Consult with fitness trainers, dietitians, and healthcare providers for personalized advice and assistance throughout your journey.

- **Fitness Apps:** Utilize fitness apps and tracking tools to monitor your progress, record workouts, and stay organized.

- **Online Communities:** Join online fitness communities or local fitness groups to connect with like-minded individuals for motivation, advice, and support.

- **Regular Progress Tracking:** Continuously assess and adapt your program as you progress. This ensures that your program remains aligned with your evolving needs and aspirations.

- **Lifelong Learning:** Stay curious and remain open to learning about new fitness techniques, nutrition trends, and holistic well-being practices.

- **Regular Check-Ins:** Schedule regular check-ins with a fitness trainer or healthcare professional to monitor your progress and adapt your program as needed.

- **Goal Setting:** Continually set new goals for yourself. Goals provide direction and motivation as you progress on your fitness journey.

- **Variety and Fun:** Keep your fitness routine fresh and enjoyable. Experiment with new exercises, activities, and wellness practices to prevent monotony and maintain your enthusiasm.

- **Community Support:** Join local fitness groups, online communities, or seek out a workout buddy. Surrounding yourself with supportive individuals can boost motivation and accountability.

- **Professional Assessment:** Periodically undergo a comprehensive assessment to gauge your overall health, evaluate your fitness progress, and refine your long-term goals.

Conclusion

As you step onto the path to your best shape, remember that this journey is an ongoing adventure. The principles of customization, personalization, and safety should always be at the forefront of your efforts. Dedication, curiosity, and the embrace of your individuality are your guiding stars.

Your best shape is not a destination but a continuous pursuit of well-being. Your commitment to this pursuit is your most valuable asset.

Stay committed, stay curious, and make each day a step toward your best shape.

About The Author

Chris G. Wenchell, a multifaceted talent in the world of entertainment and fitness, has a writing style that is not only informative but also engaging, making complex fitness concepts accessible to a wide range of readers. Chris has harnessed a lifetime of dedication to wellness to create "90 Days to Your Best Shape: A Science-Based Fitness Transformation." With a passion for physical fitness that has spanned decades, Chris brings a unique blend of personal experience, expertise, and a genuine desire to help others achieve their peak physical potential.

From an early age, Chris has been immersed in the world of fitness. At just 16, while many were enjoying leisurely lunches in high school, Chris made the conscious choice to hit the gym with his brother, Matt. This simple decision ignited a lifelong journey into the realms of strength, health, and body transformation.

Beyond his dedication to personal fitness, Chris has also ventured into the business side of the industry. He established an online fitness store, which has evolved into a one-stop destination for fitness enthusiasts. This store offers a carefully curated selection of workout equipment, sportswear, supplements, and recovery equipment, embodying Chris's commitment to promoting a holistic approach to well-being.

The foundation of his book, "90 Days to Your Best Shape," is rooted in both personal experience and scientific principles. By fusing these elements, they provide readers with a structured and evidence-based roadmap to achieving their fitness goals. Whether you're a beginner taking your first steps toward a healthier lifestyle or a seasoned fitness enthusiast striving for your peak, Chris's book offers comprehensive guidance and motivation.

With a genuine desire to share his wealth of knowledge and experience, Chris aspires to inspire others on their own fitness journeys. "90 Days to Your Best Shape: A Science-Based Fitness Transformation" is a testament to his unwavering dedication to helping individuals transform their lives, one workout at a time.

www.ingramcontent.com/pod-product-compliance
Lightning Source LLC
Chambersburg PA
CBHW050839260726
48660CB00006B/2338